Multiple Sclerosis and Hematopoietic Stem Cell Transplant; One Patients Journey

Nicole Corry

ISBN:1508474141
ISBN-13:978-1508474142

DEDICATION

This book is dedicated to my partner Phill, and my family, who mean the world to me

CONTENTS

Forward

By
Dr Colin J Andrews
Neurologist- Canberra Australia

This is the most moving account of a determined patient with Multiple Sclerosis going through the process of being accepted and then having autologous bone marrow transplantation performed at the Canberra Hospital.

When I read this I nearly came to tears because of her sheer courage and determination despite dealing with an illness which is associated with fatigue, pain and reduced mobility.

The section dealing with the lack of empathy she experienced from the medical profession plus also the nursing staff was certainly a lot of my patients have expressed to me and is expressed well I this book.

Not only is it very accurate in what she has mapped out, but anyone undergoing this procedure would benefit from reading this to know what is involved.

Having this procedure of course is not a picnic and this is borne out in the step-by-step account of the process Nicole Had to endure.

The end results, however, justify the procedure and I would highly recommend this being made widely available to anyone contemplating this procedure.

Fortunately the procedure is now becoming much more accepted in neurological circles and this trend is obviously going to continue.

Congratulations to Nicole for a superb account of her HSCT journey.

ACKNOWLEDGMENTS

I wish to acknowledge the following persons for the support and inspiration to create this journey, and who helped make the events in my life into a book. Firstly Ms Carmel Turner, who gave me the strength to pursue and seek treatment. Carmel is the shining light to many with Multiple Sclerosis and is an unsung hero. Secondly, Dr Colin J Andrews, for believing in me, and standing firm with his conviction to help others, and leading the way in effective treatment in Australia

1 INTRODUCTION

Firstly I should introduce myself. I am a fifty year old Australian woman with who has undergone an Autologous Hematopoietic Stem Cell Transplant for Multiple Sclerosis in Australia. I was one of a select few to undergo this treatment in the Canberra Public Hospital on the 25th of January 2011. This is my story.

It is best to start at the beginning, which is difficult as MS is an insidious disease that sneaks up on you. The first symptoms I can recall were migraines in one or both eyes, that occurred on and off from my early twenties. The migraines were later diagnosed as optic neuritis, a classic symptom, and often the first symptom of MS. But at the time I was busy raising three children and working fulltime as a Registered Nurse Night Manager at a busy rural hospital in NSW. I didn't have time to be sick, or to think too much about the odd migraine or tingly bits.

I started to develop left leg weakness and fatigue. What did I expect, I tried to rationalize that I worked nights, was overweight and not young anymore, so of course I was wearing down a bit. My domestic life was also in turmoil, trying to meet everyone's needs in my own and immediate family. My marriage broke down and I was sharing custody with three now teenage children with my ex-husband.

Eventually, I went to see my family Doctor about the 'bloody leg pain' in my hip that was causing me to drag my left leg a bit. The family doctor, who had seen me through pregnancies and illness, did a gross neurological examination. His look of concern told me there was a lot more going on than a 'crook hip'.

2 DIAGNOSIS

So began the conveyor belt of scans, tests and physical examinations that would soon take over my normal life. It is a frightening time in anyone's life, the waiting period between tests and results. This is often called 'limbo' and is most unsettling when you know something is wrong, but you don't know what. My mind was racing from bad to worse and back again. Was it a stroke, a brain tumor or what? My new partner Phill was a great support at this worrying time.

MS is usually diagnosed, alongside clinical presentation (that is, what you look like, can you walk, do you have tremor or other symptoms) as well as a battery of scans, head and spinal CTs and MRI's. medical procedures include lumbar puncture and evoked potential tests and EEG's. It felt like I had undergone every test known to man. The large amount of investigation is required to exclude other conditions and narrow down the possibilities of other diseases. I remember going to pathology to have my initial blood work done and telling the receptionist that I wanted 'One of everything'. It certainly felt like that at the time.

As I live in a small rural town, the wait for appointments even for initial consultations can be long. Specialists are few and far between and the time form referral to consult can be lengthy. Then on to the scanning or further testing, all the while trying to maintain your composure while working and worrying. This time took its toll on me, and I became increasingly frustrated when multiple examinations and differential diagnoses where mentioned.

One minute I was queried having a stroke, due to left leg weakness, another possible diagnosis was some sort of hereditary paralysis. All this waiting and multiple examinations are also to rule out other illness and diseases, but I have empathy for others making the same journey. Eventually a diagnosis is made.

I was about to undergo a reality shock. The visiting neurologist told us that I had Multiple Sclerosis, most likely primary progressive. There was no treatment or cure for the type of MS I had. Within ten years I would most likely be in a wheelchair or bedbound, certainly lose my employment and most likely my relationship.

The neurologist also didn't want to see me again as there was nothing he could do for me. The date, Friday 3d January 2006 is burned into my memory as the turning point in my life. This person had destroyed my whole world with this news, and had shown no empathy or even a ray of hope. I was devastated, and the walls had started closing in on me.

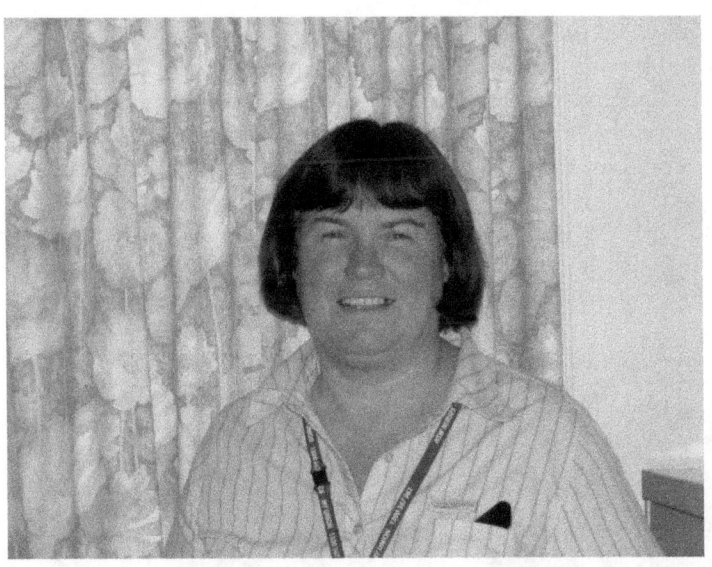

Keeping up a brave face despite failing health and unknown diagnosis.

.

That Doctor had not taken into consideration one thing. I was not just another patient. After a few days of wallowing in grief and self-pity, I gathered my strength and started to fight back for my life. I was an intelligent, educated and strong woman, with an understanding of health and the healthcare system. I went into overdrive researching my condition and current therapies as well as treatments, talking to experts and other patients in an attempt to understand the disease and help myself.

I joined the local MS Support Group, who really helped me to navigate through the maze if things I needed to know and understand. This illness, like many others, doesn't come with a manual. The group helped me through the Centrelink minefield, and explained about the various disability payments, travel schemes and allowances for financial support.

I needed a disability parking permit, and the group told me not to be stressed about applying for one as 'they give them out like lollies' at the roads and traffic centre. One of the members also encouraged me to apply for the mobility allowance, an allowance that helps with transport costs while I was still working. This allowance is not means tested. Advice and support made a big difference, but so did the friendliness of the group.

One of the more difficult concepts initially, was the fact that as my disease progressed, my leg strength and balance deteriorated, and I needed help. Walking became difficult and I fatigued easily. Especially in the heat. I needed to consider aids. Firstly I refused the offer of a walking stick, until I realized how much it helped, both with balance and distance. I wasn't keen,

3

but it soon became an indispensible part of my life

The mobility scooter was much more difficult, as I didn't want to make that decision. Eventually I purchased a Liberty mobility scooter. This scooter is able to be folded up and put in the boot of my car. Very convenient, I could manage this myself. It was also airline suitable, and we took it everywhere, but it just seemed to me to be one step closer to not walking. One heartless person saw me on my first outing on the scooter and said loudly 'what do you need that for, you can walk'. Yes, I could still walk, about two hundred yards, not the length of the shopping centre with my groceries!

www.libertymobilityaids.com.au

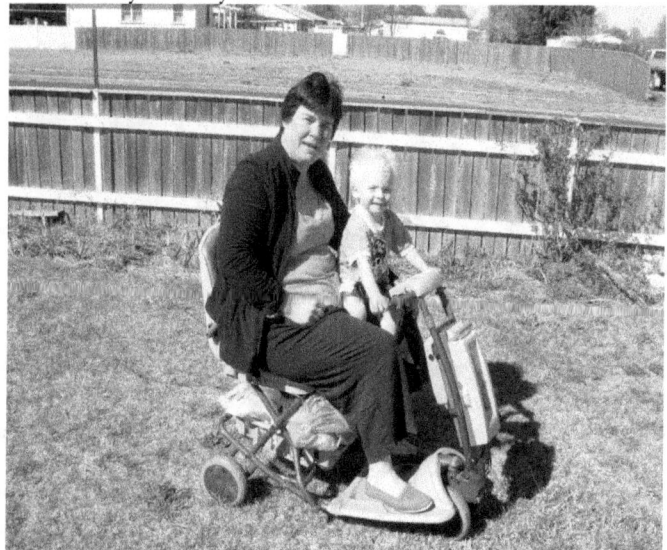

Pictured here with my grandson Brent, who wanted to drive nana's scooter.

My leg left pain and ongoing muscle spasms were a concern, so my GP proceeded to prescribe me a muscle relaxant, commonly used by MS patients to relieve the muscular spasms and cramps. This was all well and good, the medication was an inexpensive pill to be taken twice a day. However the dose is meant to be gradually increased in small steps. After one day at the 'usual' dose, I was unable to stay awake, let alone get out of bed or walk! Oops, better try a smaller dose to start.............

Interestingly, every person with MS I met seemed to be on a different medication. There didn't seem to be a 'Gold standard' of treatment.

3 DISCLOSURE

As a healthcare worker, I soon felt ostracized in the workplace. I had become the nurse with 'the dreaded MS' and felt more like a patient than a colleague. Many of the medical staff I had worked alongside had failed to recognize what must seem now, like obvious symptoms. One orthopedic surgeon asked if he could help with my now obvious limp. When I told him thanks, but you can't help, I have MS, he stated that that I made him feel like a right bastard for asking me!

Disclosing to my Director of Nursing was a difficult decision to make, but I felt it had to be done promptly as my symptoms were worsening. The response I received, after over twenty plus years' service was 'well, you will be leaving then?' No empathy from this HealthCARE manager.

I did not leave, but reskilled several times to maintain employment and an income. Very limited assistance came from the organization, considering I worked in health. Nothing came easily and everything was a battle. Phill was at UNE completing his Bachelor of Nursing and I felt pressured to continue working, both for an income and my self-esteem. I didn't know until later that I would become defined by who I was, not the job I did.

The position that I held at that time was as a Transport Nurse with the Internal Patient Transport team attached to the hospital. Our role was to provide non urgent transport across our region. It was a dream job. The driver Warren was a kind and considerate man, who I am still friends with today. As part of a team, when my symptoms became obvious, it was hard to leave that situation and move on. Knowing when to do that is hard, and its takes personal strength to admit that it's time to let go. I'm sure it's just as hard for others watching me deteriorate as well, and frustrating when they can't help.

4 THE SURPRISE TRIP

I joined the society that assists people with Multiple Sclerosis in Australia. The society provides a wealth of information and support services, especially to the newly diagnosed, their families and carers. MS Australia co–ordinates many programs, such as the well-known MS readathon and the Sydney to Wollongong fun run as well as many other projects. The organization also provides many networks such as peer support, they offer a newly diagnosed program, counseling, a reference library and produce an informative quarterly information magazine. The Society also contributes significantly to Australian research, and has links to social media and runs webinars as well as one on one telephone counseling support. Basically they are all over it.

www.ms.org.au

The society also provides a Nurse for one on one support, education and training. While this is very beneficial, the rural area I live in is vast and a lot of time is spent travelling to see clients. The Nurse also attends the support group and is available via telephone contact as well for clients nd families.

The Society also provides scholarships to assist persons with MS to achieve their dreams. MS Australia run a 'Go for Gold' scholarship each year. Several categories are available, such as travel, education and the arts. In 2007 I secretly applied in the travel category. My dream was to take my partner Phill on a trip to Tasmania. This trip of a lifetime would give us the opportunity to spend some time travelling while I was still able to walk short distances. I wanted to give back to Phill..

It was a big ask to take on a diagnosis like MS in your partner. We had not been together very long when this happened, and Phill did not hesitate to provide me with support and reassurance. Not many people would selflessly put their hand up under these circumstances.

I showed Phill the application that I had already submitted. He said it might need more work. It was too late, we had won! Included in the scholarship were flights to Melbourne to attend the award dinner and a conference.

The award dinner and conference were a real eye opener. We got to meet a lot of the team behind MS Australia, and see first-hand what a large organization it is. We watched a lot of presentations and met some of the previous award winners.

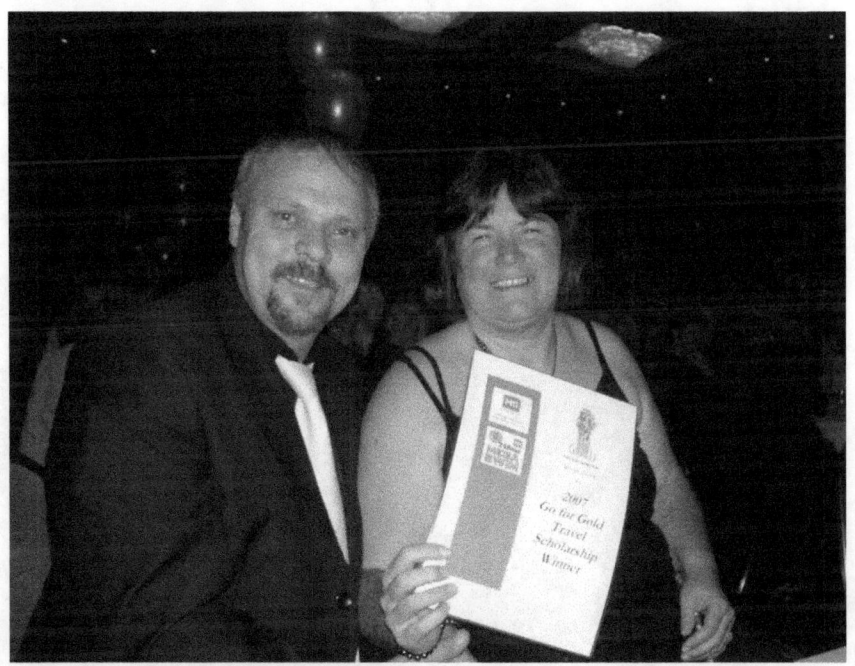
Phill and myself at the 2007 awards dinner in Melbourne

Phill and I went to the conference the next day after the award dinner. There were a lot of people with MS attending, and it was too much for Phill, he had to go for a long walk. I was also distressed at the number of people with MS, especially the severity of the disease in young people.

Around my table were people trying to make sense of their lives, and I especially remember one woman like myself, who was too scared to disclose to her employer about her illness. I felt for her not wanting to disclose after my own awful experience. I was starting to see the big picture, and how many Australians were affected.

What a fantastic time we had in Tasmania! Despite having limited mobility, and having to cart the scooter everywhere with us, Tassie is a great spot to visit. Most places were wheelchair friendly, and the locals went out of their way to make both of us feel welcome. I would strongly advise using a travel agent when going with a wheelchair or limited mobility, as you can avoid disappointment if you can't access places. The travel agent we used made our trip go smoothly with the benefit of their experience.

However, we did go 'off road' a couple of times. Once at Cataract Gorge in Launceston, where the scooter battery just made the distance on the walking path into the gorge. We also did the night ghost tour at Port Arthur, thanks to a couple of burley men, and a great guide. The countryside was beautiful, and we made the most of the trip, thinking it may be our last. While we were away, my family had set to work making our house more accessible and applying long needed finishing touches to the kitchen.. I am very grateful for the love and support mum and Bill have always shown me, and of course big sister Donna.

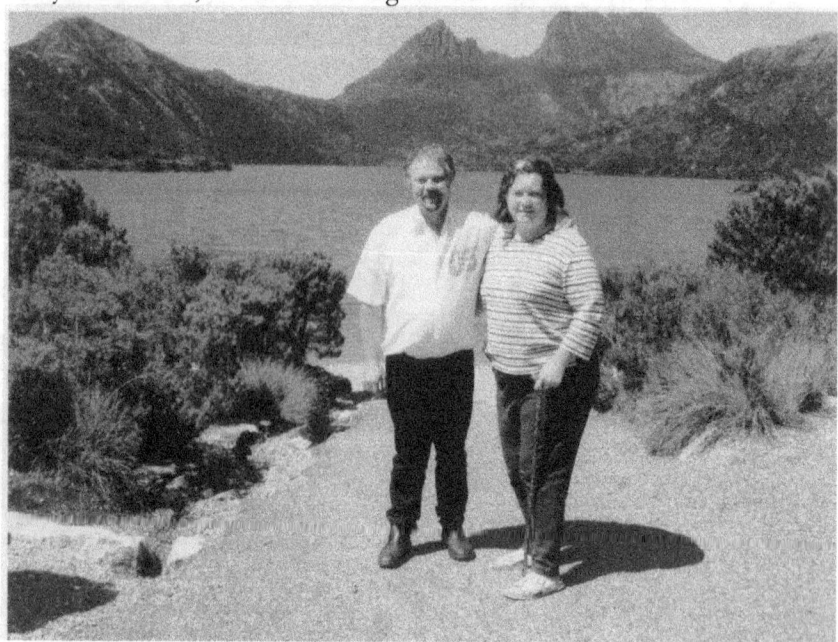

Cradle mountain in Tasmania 2007

5 BACK TO WORK

Back to work. It was if I had never been away. The work minefield intesified as I quickly worsened, needing a walking stick, then a motorised scooter to get around the large distance of hospital corridoors. The jump to taking the scooter to work was a big one. I felt embarrassed that I needed it, but the distances of the walking were getting beyond me. If I needed to carry anything, like store or medical records, I just couldn't do it. Hospital staff soon got used to seeing me on it, but I was never really comfortable about it.

I was now employed as a Ward Clerk, and the work was much more physically demanding than I had anticipated. Going from a Registered Nurse position to Ward Clerk was difficult and financially crippling. When you change jobs, even in the same organization, everything is affected. All my accrued leave was now under the lower pay classification. Staff attitudes changed as well. Boundaries had to be constantly reset as I established my new role. There is only one clerk in the busy Accident and Emergency department, with no relief for busy times, or even lunch.

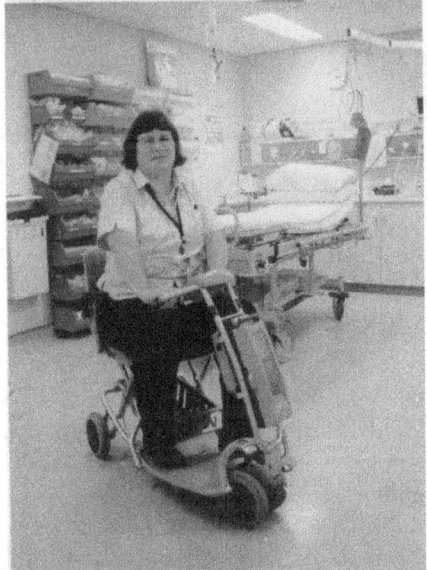

No consideration was given to any workplace modifications or system changes to make the workplace more accommodating, despite requests. So I battled on, and found a place to park my scooter that wasn't 'in everybody's way'. Exhaustion and pain were constant companions during the day, and increased at night, making sleeping almost impossible. My time driving home from work was mainly spent crying, so I could compose myself and put on a brave face when I got home.

An unexpected release from that time came in 2008, when a work colleague from Community Health suggested that I should apply for a position that was available in their team. As I had already worked in the position on a secondment in the past for a few months, I already knew the role. I applied and was successful. The position was a management role, office orientated, managing a team of allied health professionals. The job came with increased responsibilities and a substantial pay increase. I would have my own office and much better working conditions. The office was also on the second floor of a building with no lift....

However in true Nicole Corry style, I was being assessed in Brisbane for a 'Walkaide'. This electrical nerve stimulating device was new in Australia at that time. After being fitted with the device by the consultant, the device was calibrated to my individual walking gait. The Walkaide worked well enough that I could walk the distances needed in my new role , and even up stairs! Expensive and not painless, this little heard of device helped with my leg swelling and footdrop as well as gait improvement.

These devices are commonly called FES or functional electronic stimulation devices. This aid could be helping a large amount of people with MS and the associated footdrop. I had to source the product and supplier myself, luckily the consultant was in Australia and running a clinic.

The Walkaide works externally, the patient places the electrode on the skin over the superficial peroneal nerve on the outside of the affected leg around the knee area, and turns on the device. As the patient walks, the device senses the rhythm and paces the foot to lift. Once calibrated, I had a much greater use of my foot and improved walking gait, speed and distance. Battery operated and easily concealed under my clothes, it was a real bonus to keep me mobile.

www.Walkaide.com

With the change of job, my working life had been extended yet again, but my left leg was wasting and becoming stiff. My legs would go into painful muscular spasms, and I began to need my walking stick most of the time now. I would plan my tasks for the day and think ahead to ensure the most efficient use of walking. For example, visit the bathroom and collect the mail on the way back, and co-ordinate my trips downstairs to do several tasks.

I worked hard and enjoyed the time I spent working with the Community Health team. I felt valued and supported. My physical limitations meant that the day was long, but I paced myself and kept on top of things. Typing was reduced to one hand most days, as the creeping numbness was now extending to my hands as well, and they were becoming weak and painful. I was surprised to receive a huge vote of confidence from the team when I was presented with employee of the month in June 2009. However I was still grinding downwards and my working days were numbered. Credit must go to the General Manager Wendy, who threatened to 'drag me to work I a wheelchair if she had to'. The day was looming though, and after a fall at work, I resigned in late 2009, nearly a year later.

I sought financial advice prior to leaving employment, and was lucky to have TPD or total and permanent disability insurance. Warning to the unwary, seek finance advice before you leave work, as there are many pitfalls and this can mean huge difference financially. Most superannuation schemes have TPD built in, if you are unaware and collect your superannuation, your insurance is void.

I had never even been inside Centrelink. As a fulltime employee my entire working life, I had never needed to go there. The process of applying for benefits seemed endless, and the information required kept me busy for quite some time. The GP had to sign off on my illness and then we went through the third degree on my ability to work. I had a work capacity assessment, where I told the assessor that I had reskilled three times to remain employed, before I simply could not work anymore. The physical assessment was pretty short..

I was granted the Disability support pension, and remember wondering how on earth we were going to survive. Phill was granted the carers allowance and pension, and was working a few nights a week to supplement our income when he could. Working also gave Phill a badly needed outlet from 24/7 care.

6 RETIREMENT

In retirement my condition worsened and depression set in. My world had become very small and I was lonely, used to the hum of an active working life. I was at home by myself a lot of the time. I had chronic pain, day in and day out, and would be screaming in pain at night.

My hands were just useless in strength, and my fine motor skills were poor. It was getting to the point that I couldn't cook or carry a cup of coffee without risking injury.

Nowhere is mentioned the grief that I felt from slowly losing my life. I was losing my body image, my sense of self, and the strength the of person I was. I felt like I was disappearing. I refer to this as my 'cloak of disability'. Whenever I went out, especially on the scooter, people would either not make eye contact or look right through me. Discussions would be held over my head like I wasn't there. If I got angry, I would remind people that I was physically disabled, not mentally. A small bonus, I was never asked to buy raffle tickets!

Phill would help dress me for the day, as shoes and buttons were becoming difficult. Phill also took on other roles when needed, assisting in daily tasks such as helping me wash my hair and run hot water, as I could not feel the temperature of the water. I despaired that I was turning into a patient, rather than his partner. Fatigue and heat were huge concerns, and I feared that I was sleeping my life away.

I had nothing to do all day and was becoming self-absorbed. I researched and chatted online with MS sufferers. I needed to regain some sense of self and control in my life. I looked toward my community for support and activities. Work 'friends' had faded away apart from two or three, who are still in touch today. I needed an interest and volunteering was the way to go. The Saint Vincent de Paul Guyra Centre was a great outlet. I felt valued and welcome when I was well enough to attend. This gave me a link to my local community, enabled me to make friends with local women, and gave me an outlet (and Phill got a break too).

7 STEM CELL AND OTHER THERAPIES

Not long after I had retired from work, I saw an article in treating Multiple Sclerosis with autologous stems cells in Germany. The Xcell Centre in Cologne, Germany, were accepting overseas patients.

Phill and I read about the treatment they were offering. We spoke to the representative and patients who had been treated at the centre. I applied for treatment and was accepted. I did not undertake this step lightly, as once again there was a financial cost as well as an emotional input. A lot of discussion, soul searching and consideration went into deciding to go outside Australia for treatment.

The XCell Centre was licensed and accredited by the Geman government. I am aware that there is a large amount of negativity regarding medical tourism and going overseas for treatment. It the treatment is not available in your country, and there was the possibility of effective treatment outside of Australia, could you honestly say you would not go? If it was your partner, your child or someone you cared about, wouldn't you want them to have help if it was on offer?

I was accepted for treatment, and we booked to fly to Germany for Autologous Stem Cell Therapy in late 2009. Passports in hand, we travelled half way around the world with my trusty wheelchair scooter to have autologous stem cell therapy. I might sound desperate, or clutching at straws, but I firmly believe that you need to take your health into your own hands and fight. I have one life, and I wanted to live it.

A warning about airports, if you need assistance, be early, polite and courteous. Once your wheelchair or aid is booked in, the airport staff need to be able to assist you and have a wheelchair booked. Being disabled doesn't mean you board first. Be polite and patient, as you will usually be seated after everyone else have boarded and the staff have time to assist you. Special requirements need to be made at time of booking, not when running late for a flight..

I find it funny now, although I didn't then, that the fat lady in the wheelchair ALWAYS gets searched. Make sure you are organized and have all your paperwork, Dr's letters and medications at the ready. I always allow plenty of time to get through the checkouts and allow time for that last cigarette if Phill is going..

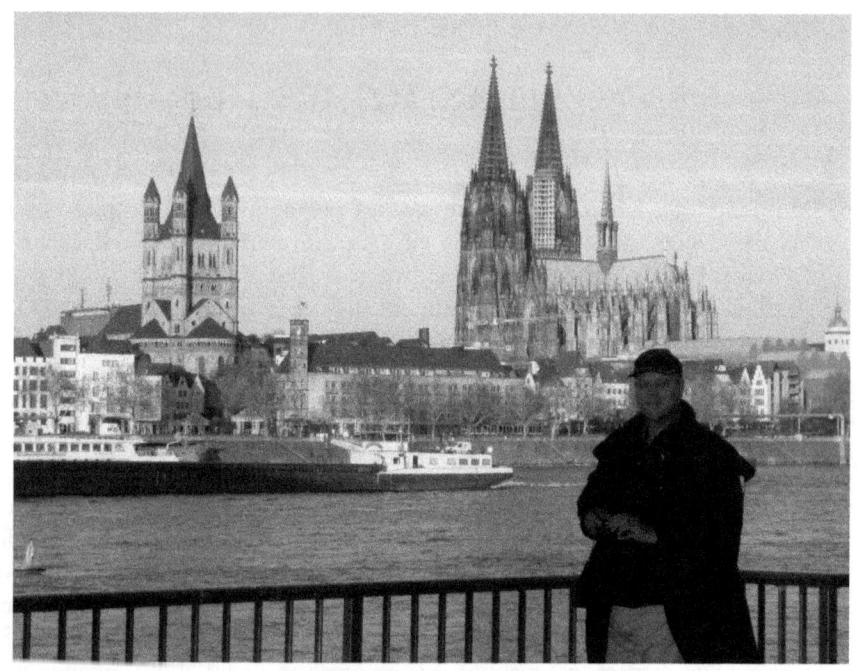

Phill in Cologne, Germany, 2009

On the twenty fourth of November 2009 I underwent the stem cell treatment under the guidance of the experienced medical staff at the XCell centre. The Autologous stem cell treatment consisted of simple bone marrow aspiration, filtering out the stem cells and reinjection into the patient. No chemotherapy was used in this therapy. The bone marrow aspiration was under local anesthetic and was extremely painful. We were away a week at huge personal and financial expense.

Did it work? While I felt improved for a short while, it did provide me with something else that had been lacking for a long time. Hope. That somewhere out there, stem cell related research was close to an effective treatment. If not for me, then others diagnosed with this cruel, painful, debilitating slow death. I liken it to suffocating in slow motion quicksand.

Addit; Licensed by the German government, the XCell centre ceased operation in 2011.

As well as the German stem cell treatment, I had tried both electrical and physical aids. I purchased a MOTOmed movement therapy system, walking and other exercise equipment to prevent muscle wastage. Regular visits to the physiotherapist and hydrotherapy were also on the agenda. As word spread, unsolicited advice abounded, and I feel that I have heard every theory on causation and cure, from bee venom to goat serum and back again. My mother also offered her standard sage advice 'perhaps if I lost some weight...............' The obvious cure for everything in life!

I don't have a personal dieting philosophy, everyone that I know seems to be on a perpetual diet. If it helps you, great. I find eating one of the great pleasures in life, and I have seen others swear by prescription diets. Sorry, not me.

Treatments abound, and no two persons with MS seem to be on the same regime. I tried all the pharmaceutical treatments available trying to slow the progression of my disease down. I injected myself with 'easy to use' spring loaded devices containing immunomodulation drugs. These simply made me feel worse and caused huge hard lumps no matter where they were injected. I also had an automated device which came with a drug company nurse to instruct me on its use, all the way from Sydney. This drug caused 'mild flu like symptoms.' Yeah right, fever and rigor more like after every dose, so that was short-lived. Why take an expensive drug to make you sicker?

Infusions consisted of high dose prednisone, and Mitoxantrone and Tysabri, all of whom have their own nasty side effects. Nothing seemed to make any difference in the pain, weakness or progression. My mind had started to become confused and conversations sometimes drifted away and I would lose the train of what I was saying. I could not hold a sensible conversation or stay on topic. Things were looking grim.

8 IN THE MEANTIME

It has to be acknowledged that all this hoping, researching and trying new therapies is hard, emotionally, physically and financially. MS doesn't affect one person; it affects a whole family and ripples outward. My partner Phill and family have weathered the highs and lows, and still have to tend to the everyday things. The world doesn't stop when someone is sick, and I had now been sick for a number of years. Simple things like shopping and paying the bills still have to be done and life rolls on.

Sometimes, when it's all too much and I get angry, I think I would like one day without pain. MS is everyday, there's no day off for you or anyone else around you. It's easy to get frustrated and upset. I see the effect this has on those I love around me and it spurs me on to appreciate all that I do have, not what I don't. This positive attitude serves me well. I call this benefit sense. It means looking at what you can do, not what you can't.

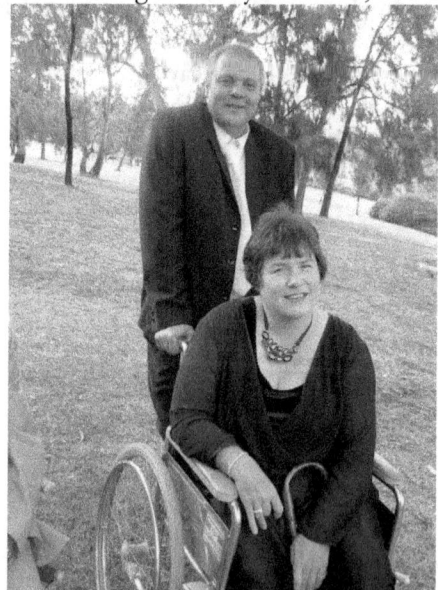

Phill and myself at Donnas wedding.

In March 2010 my beautiful sister Donna married Craig Montgomery. Craig and his family became part of ours. Craig and Donna were a big part of my support network, and it must be said that without family and friends, I would never have gotten as far as I did in my search for an effective treatment. I realize how precious life is and value those around me who show they care. It's not easy to watch a family member struggle.

The wedding was held at the Armidale Arboretum, a beautiful outdoors wedding. However it was too far and too steep for me to walk, so I had to use a wheelchair to attend. The day was beautiful, only marred by a relative commenting on the fact that many of the people that I used to work with that attended did not take the time to say hello to me. 'Don't you know all those people?' yes I did, but that was another lifetime ago…

I continued to search far and wide for the latest in treatments and research. We travelled to Sydney to The Brain, Mind and Research institute to be seen by 'the top MS professor and principal researcher in Australia' who promptly told me there was nothing new for my form of MS and he 'didn't even know why I was here'. I told him I wished to be flagged as a willing participant in any new clinical trials that may become available in Australia. I would not just curl up at home like I have seen others do.

I sought many different opinions and read widely on international treatments, as well as clinical trials worldwide. It must be noted that the patient community is global. I can easily communicate with people in Russia, Tunisia and India. I can access any information on virtually any subject in multiple medias, such as websites, forums, blogs. Patients can be well informed, if they choose to be.

My search led me to Newcastle, to be examined for the possibility of CCSVI (Chronic cerebrospinal venous insufficiency) I underwent a duplex untrasound of the extracranial veins in my neck. There is mounting evidence that venous insufficiency in some people diagnosed with MS exists. When treated for an existing abnormality, the person's symptoms improve. This endovascular treatment has been pioneered by Dr Paollo Zamboni, University of Ferrara, Italy.

www.CCSVIAustralia.com for more information

I personally feel that if any person demonstrates an area of vascular abnormality, low venous flow, occlusion or stenosis, they have every right to be treated. I also feel that this type of demonstrated venous insufficiency in MS population warrants a serious rethink of the classification of Multiple Sclerosis. Is there a venous cause within the defined population? More exploration on this area is required.

After the ultrasound I was referred to St Vincents Hospital in Sydney, and underwent a jugular venogram on the twenty ninth of October 2010. After having the venogram, and building my hopes up, the Doctor performing the procedure told me 'sorry, we can't help you'. It was a real low point.

All the grief that had been collecting inside me just let go. The fighting and trying seemed hopeless, and I dissolved into a crying, screaming wreck as complete anguish washed over me. This episode didn't last long, but sure did upset the day surgery nurse! Back to square one.

9 STEM CELL THERAPY IN AUSTRALIA

As I was interested in stem cell therapy, and felt it was the direction that MS treatment would take, I learned of a young man, Ben Leahy, via an ABC news segment *Miracle Recovery* 2008. This young man was in Australia and had been treated with Autologous stem cells. His recovery was amazing. At the same time internationally, Dr Richard Burt and colleagues at Northwestern University in Chicago were conducting an early phase study on Autologous Hematopoietic Stem cell Transplantation. The results were encouraging, and further trials are being run.

Then things really started to happen for me. Funny thing, the next big breakthrough came not from any medical study or journal, but from a national women's magazine. The 'New Idea' had an article featuring a lady called Carmel Turner and was tilted Miracle MS Cure. Well, I was on fire, hope rekindled and I was on a mission.

I contacted Carmel and found her to be a guiding light. This woman gives up so much of her time to help people with MS and their families it's amazing. Carmel spent time listening to me and advising me in my search for answers and treatment. Carmel has opened up her life on a website to provide much needed knowledge and first –hand information.

http://msstemcell.com./Home.php

Carmel gave me the contact details and advice on applying to the Canberra specialist who treated her. I rang to see if I could get a consultation. The specialist centre sent out guidelines on the criteria they used to see if I met their criteria to be considered for treatment. All I needed now was a referral from the local Neurologist! Sounds easy.

The local Neurologist was not keen to give me a referral, citing that I wouldn't be accepted, and even if it did work, it would come back twice as bad. Oh and the risk of death was high. Not to be put off, I asked for a referral, not his opinion. Referral in hand, I was on my way, off to Canberra.

We live in Guyra, rural New South Wales on the new England Highway. It's a sleepy little town where most people are friendly and I feel at home. It's also ten hours by car to Canberra. Off we go, fearful and hopeful at the same time. I have read as much as I can, but it's all up to the Doctor we are about to see. We arrive tired at the Canberra Hospital residences, book in and prepare for our appointment the next day.

Phill and I arrive at the Canberra Specialist Medical Centre in plenty of time for my appointment, and I have every scan and test result I have with us. I was feeling nauseous with hope and anticipation. We walk into the centre and I'm trying to look my best as we wait to be seen. I'm as nervous as hell. On the wall were Carmel and Ben Leahy's media releases. I'm in the right place!

I finally get to meet Dr Colin J Andrews. We are ushered into his rooms and Dr Andrews begins to get a feel for my condition and questions me closely on current as well as past treatments and symptoms. He reads my referral and scan results and does a lengthy clinical examination. Thing's aren't good. Dr Andrews needs more information (Blast!) and refers me for yet more enhanced scans and an infusion of Mitoxantrone. Well at least I'm in his sights.

So back on the therapy and scans conveyor belt, and we await the outcome of yet another MRI's with enhancement and my response to another round of Mitoxantrone. A word to the unwary, make sure your radiology is licensed with Medicare for MRI's. Ours wasn't and there was no rebate to claim. A huge out of pocket expense that is unnecessary.

Phill and I went to stay at his sister Ruth's house in Nowra, thankfully a close haven. Ruth and her husband Frank have been a real blessing, always welcoming and ready to help. Ruth is one of life's gems. She doesn't know how special she is.

Scan done, and infusion completed, we head home for a few weeks. I consult with Carmel, who encourages me to be strong and think positive. I have a good result from the Mitoxantrone, with my symptoms settling down a bit. While we are waiting, I resolve to sell myself as a good candidate for the stem cell treatment, known as HSCT.

Hematopoietic stem cell transplant has been around for more than a decade, but is not an approved treatment for Multiple Sclerosis. When applied to MS cases, it is viewed as experimental and the long term benefits are yet to be proven. As stated previously, I only have one life, and I couldn't wait around for a decade or so until the powers that be decide it might be safe.

10 THE TRANSPLANT COUNTDOWN

Phill and I return to Canberra, quietly hopeful. As we wait for my appointment, I feel confident but nervous. I present myself as an informed candidate, with family and financial support. We go into Dr Andrews office and I proceeded to sell myself as a candidate for HSCT. I had nothing to lose and a life to gain. It was the biggest chance of my life. Another round of questions and examinations and then finally the big decision, would I be accepted?

Yes! On condition that the Canberra Ethics Committee was as sold on my need for this type of treatment. I was in. I didn't know it at the time, but the treatment program was I jeopardy of closing due to objections by some of the committee. I would be the seventh patient to undergo HSCT at the Canberra Hospital.

Home to Guyra to await scheduling for treatment. As transplant involves the Neurology department, Hematology and Oncology, the therapy needs major organization and liaison for the admission and treatment of a patient. The Transplant Nurse would co-ordinate the specialties and advise us of the plan of treatment and chemo dates.

We would need to stay near the hospital as an outpatient while I had chemotherapy. We had to search around and look at our options as it was a long way from home. Thankfully we were eligible to stay in the Canberra Residences at the hospital. The cost was upfront, with a rebate from the Isolated Patients Travel Assistance Scheme, IPTASS. The scheme provides rebates for eligible patients and their carers who need to travel to access treatment. This can include private car kilometer and accommodation allowances. The financial side of things was going to be tough, and we would have to rely on family support to enable me to undergo the treatment.

So began the real journey towards HSCT. I had an appointment with the treating Hematologist. The specialist was a very pleasant and thorough Doctor, who went over the procedure in-depth with Phill and myself, and also with the Transplant Nurse. It was good to put a face to the person who had been orchestrating all of my care.

The Nurse took me to the Apheresis Unit, where all the action would happen, and answered my myriad of questions. I also completed another health screen, which included a total skin and body check, mucosal membranes and dental health. These strict examinations prior to commencement ensure that the patient is in the best condition, and has no possible sources of infection such as tooth decay. I toured the

Chemotherapy day ward, which operates every day and treats a large volume of patients. I was amazed at how efficiently and smoothly the ward ran. It is a credit to the hard working staff.

Stem cell mobilization is when peripheral blood stem cells are harvested from the blood stream, and are stored for reinfusion at a later time, usually frozen. Stem cells are normally found in bone marrow. To encourage stem cells to move from the bone marrow to the bloodstream, chemotherapy and marrow stimulating hormones are administered. Blood pathology prior to commencement of treatment is essential, and includes a full screen of the patients health, this also includes a screen for viruses.

Given a clean bill of health, I commenced day chemotherapy. I had strict instructions regarding hygiene, fever and avoiding any possible sources of infection. Phill was staying with me at this time, as I was unable to cook or look after myself. The daily chemo took its toll, and I was glad of Phill's help to do even small tasks. Finding a vein became a real challenge each day, as well as sitting for hours in one place. Nausea and fatigue kicked in, and I simply slept. Very weak, I was glad Phill was with me. I couldn't have managed being an outpatient on my own. It was very hot in Canberra at that time, and probably very boring for Phill, who had to occupy himself while I was at chemo most of the day.

Chemo done after a week or so, and it was on to the marrow stimulating hormones, or G-CSF. The marrow stimulating hormones, G-CSF or stem cell factor, commence about 24hours after chemo. The first dose is done in the clinic under supervision in case of allergic reaction. As Phill and I are both Registered Nurses, administering the twice daily subcutaneous injections was simple. Other patients would have to be shown or have the Community nurse do this. Day one and two go smoothly, I rest and potter about, waiting for pathology to collect my blood each morning to check my cell count. As the days go by, my hips, and thigh bones start to ache. It is hard to describe the feeling, but it's a good sign that collection would soon take place.

About a week later, pathology ring to say that the morning's blood count indicated that collection could be done that day! They have already booked me into the Apheresis unit this morning. It's all happening! I rushed in to tell Phill the news that the collection was going ahead that day. We made our way over to the Apheresis unit to have my stem cells collected, commonly known as harvesting.

The stem cells are collected from the bloodstream by an Apheresis machine. This occurs when the blood is separated by centrifugal force to separate the stem cells from other blood components. Prior to commencement a central line was inserted into my groin on the right hand side. Apart from the local, this wasn't painful, just uncomfortable, and it was much better than trying to find a suitable peripheral vein in my arm.

After checking the central line was patent, I was hooked up to the Apheresis unit and collection commenced. This can take several hours, and I was monitored closely. Side effects while undergoing this procedure can include breathlessness, tingling lips, fingers or feeling lightheaded. I felt a bit flush, and the nurse monitored my temperature closely. The collection took a few hours, and I had no untoward side effects.

The filtered stem cells on completion of harvesting, are mixed with DMSO, a preservative that allows the stems cells to be cryopreserved. After being cryopreserved, the stem cells can remain viable for years.

I was transferred to the ward after collection to stay overnight, planning to remove my femoral line in the morning. That all sounds organized and straightforward. Phill was waiting to pick me up when I was discharged, and the Doctor arrived and removed the femoral line. As s femoral line is a large lumen, I had to lie flat with moderate pressure on my groin puncture site for an hour. When the time was up, I tried to stand up and the site blew. Lots and lots of blood flew everywhere. I yelled out for the nurse and tried to put pressure over the puncture site. There was so much blood that I couldn't find the site to stop the bleeding. My hand pressure was also hopeless. It was truly an emergency. The nurse ran off to get help, and a Resident Doctor came to my aid and put decent pressure over the site. This frightened me, scared Phill and the nurse looking after me wasn't too keen to deal with me after that either.

After all that excitement, I ended up staying a further day as my temperature was rising on and off. After much consultation, my abdomen was scanned and it was decided that prior to transplant it would be in my best interests to have my gall bladder removed prior to further treatment. Back to Guyra to consult a surgeon.

The local GP was really positive and got me a consult rather quickly. It was now late 2011, and knowing the hospital system, most of the Doctors go on leave over the Christmas period. However, due to the fact I was awaiting transplant, and already had stem cells collected and frozen waiting, I slipped onto the one of last surgical waiting lists before the Christmas shutdown. Lucky, Lucky; Lucky.

The laparoscopic cholecystectomy was performed on the nineteenth of December 2011. I had an unremarkable overnight admission. I had my eye on the prize of getting back to Canberra and being fit to transplant. I cooled my heels at home, waiting for an admission date. I was unaware that the Ethics Committee at the Canberra Hospital were close to shutting down the program, or how truly fortunate I was to be having this treatment in Australia.

Two or three weeks after chemo I went into my bathroom at home with a scalp that felt sunburnt. As I ran my hands through my itchy scalp, my thick brown hair fell out into my hands. It all wanted to fall out at once.

The patchy clumps left were soon shaved off by Phill, until I was completely bald. I could now moisturize my itchy scalp. My nudie head was soon to be followed by the rest of my entire body hair. This really didn't worry me, as I have endured a lifetime of plucking, waxing, tweezing and shaving. I was finally hair free!

Wigs and scarves were used to cove my nudie head, and I enjoyed sharing the long wig I had purchased with my good friend Janice. Janice looked so funny with long wig on. She said she had not had long hair 'since she was a girl'. My head did get cold, but I wigs, scarves and plenty of hats to wear. My hair did grow back eventually, and the wigs and scarves were donated to the local wig library. While my hair grew back soft, it didn't grow back blonde or curly....

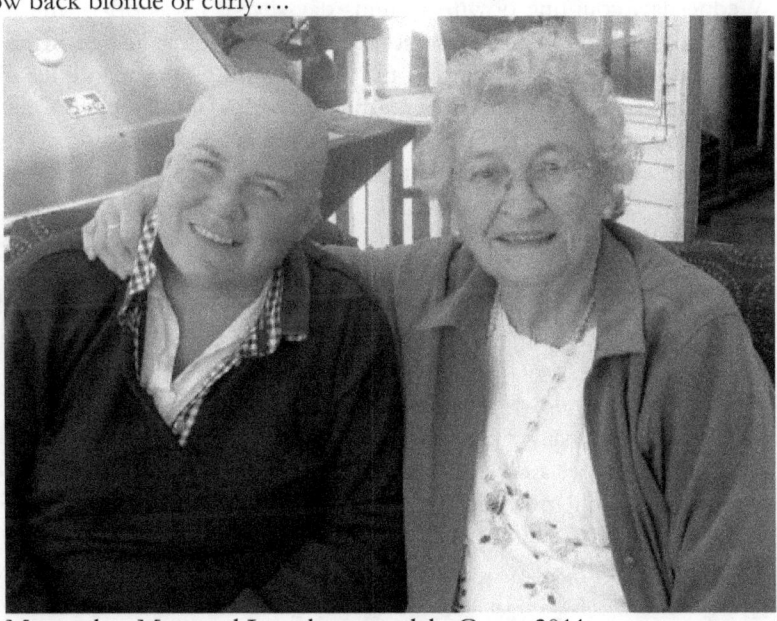

My mother Mary and I on the verandah, Guyra 2011

The call came in from the Transplant Nurse. We were to be back in Canberra on the fifteenth of January for an angiogram and insertion of a Hickman's line on the following day. Phill and I made our way back to Canberra a few days earlier and had last minute consults with both the Hematologist and Dr Andrews.

An angiogram is needed so that I could have a large intravenous line, called a Hickman's inserted into one of the large veins in my chest. This line would hopefully stay in for the rest of my treatment, and used for round of chemo and transplant. No more trying to get peripheral vein access, yay.

The procedure went smoothly, and the line site settled nicely. It took a bit of getting used to, and extra care is needed when handling the line not to disturb or dislodge it. The nurses instructed me on how to care for the line.

11.POST TRANSPLANT

My countdown to transplant started the next day. Tuesday, counting down minus day eight, I attended the Bone Marrow Transplant unit (BMT) for final review by the whole team. An electrocardiograph and bloods were taken. This was our last chance to ask questions and check details, and for the team to check inpatient admission dates and make any adjustment to the schedule. I was quietly confident and looking towards day 0, reinfusion day.

Wednesday, counting down to minus day seven, I was off to the BMT for the chemo component. This round of chemo is designed to make me neutropenic. I would soon be at the point of no return and have no immune defenses. I was entering the highest risk stage. Hopefully all the careful preparation would see me through. I was also hoping that I was mentally and emotionally ready for the ordeal that was to come.

Thursday, counting down to minus day six, back to the BMT for the days chemo, taking special care to wash my hands and keep an eye on my temperature for any sign of infection. Arrangements were I place for my admission to the acute ward later that week. Pathology were monitoring the drop in white blood cells, neutrophils, platelets, hemoglobin, as well as liver and kidney function.

Friday, counting down to minus day five, not long to go. I was still attending the BMT daily, and honestly didn't feel too bad, just really weak and drained. I appreciated Phill still looking after me and supporting me after a long day at chemo. Keeping up my spirits a long way from home was so important.

Saturday, counting down to minus four and the weekend to go. It was very quiet in the hospital and BMT unit while I underwent weekend treatment. Most chemo is scheduled during the week, so only a few people were about. Phill and I spent time driving around Canberra after chemo taking in the city views, just spending time together, as he would soon have to leave to go home.

Sunday, counting down to minus day three. I didn't yet really know or understand what I had let myself in for in the coming weeks. I feel to consider this course of treatment you must be emotionally strong and focused.

Monday, counting down to minus day two. I remain weak and listless, attending the BMT for the second last time. Phill and I have a special dinner of overlooking Lake Burley Griffin. Steamed veggies in the car to avoid other people and possible sources of infection. So romantic.

Tuesday, counting down to minus day one. Last chemo before

reinfusion, and the last night as an outpatient before weeks of solitude. I enjoy sitting outside in the cool night breeze before going to bed. It was a balmy night and excitement mingled with fear as I drifted off to sleep.

Day ZERO! Wednesday, day zero. Phill and I attend the BMT and waited as the precious stem cells were thawed. Everyone, including the staff were upbeat on that day. It was the twenty fifth of January, Australia day 2011. The routine checks that accompany transfusions were carried out, and the moment had arrived. The small gold fluid filled bag that was to become my new immune system was fed into my body. At this point some patients have had a fishy odor sensation, I didn't experience this. The infusion only took half an hour, a bit of a letdown. I was disconnected and admitted to the post- transplant acute care unit.

As I was celebrating Australia Day with my new immune system, considered to be my new birthday by many transplant recipients, my family at home were undergoing a tragedy.. My sister Donna's husband, the funny, supportive and very often politically incorrect Craig, had passed away. Craig was waiting on a transplant list also, for a new liver that never came. I could not be there for them at that time, and my heart was breaking for Donna and Craig's parents. It is with sadness now as I celebrate each passing transplant anniversary, as it is also the anniversary of remembering Craig and what he meant to our family.

The post- transplant unit, or acute care, is a multiple single room unit, where I would be isolated until the stem cell transplant took and my body started to produce new blood components. The nurse on that day put a chart up on the wall for me to see my results each day and boost my morale, and make me feel more of the process. I still didn't feel too bad, but that was about to change. Phill was to go home that afternoon. As I was an inpatient admitted to hospital, we could not financially manage if Phill was not at home working and tending to our house and animals. Reluctantly Phill left that afternoon, and my isolation and wait began. This part of my journey would just have to be done alone.

Day One. The most exciting thing that happened all day was when the nurse wrote up the day's blood results. This way I could track any improvements and be included in the process. No progress today. My blood count was still dropping and I started to feel unwell. An ATG infusion (antithymocyte globulins) was given that day. These preparations are used primarily as induction agents, that is, drugs that are given in the immediate post transfusion phase for the prevention of rejection.

Day Two, another infusion of ATG and my blood count is still dropping. For those with a medical background, results as follows, hemoglobin 111, white cell count 0.2, platelets 183, neutrophils 0. Nausea and feeling very lightheaded joined the fatigue and overwhelming desire to sleep. Any effort to move took enormous strength. Going to the ensuite was like running a marathon, I literally flopped back onto my bed, too exhausted to roll over.

As the days rolled on, my blood count continued to drop. Now at day seven, my hemoglobin was 79, white cell count 0.1, platelets 0, neutrophils 0. This count would have been pretty easy for the lab! I now required oxygen and assistance to go to the bathroom. Any activity caused extreme breathlessness. Diarrhea had begun and compounded the effort to get to the bathroom and attend to my personal hygiene. Even talking on the phone became hard. Sitting up was too much effort, so I would put the phone under my ear on the pillow. Forget sitting up to eat, I had no appetite and eating was too much effort. Chocolate milk with a straw became my main food.

Communication with loved ones so far away was so important. I desperately wanted to be there for my sister Donna, who was grieving the loss of her husband Craig. I was so weak that I would just answer the phone and tell whoever was ringing just to talk and tell me the news, as I was too breathless and fatigued to even speak for long.

The stream of Doctors rounds would happen, and the meals would come and go. The Nurses would tell me about their day and the outside world, and time drifted by. Each room on the ward had a television, and I tried to keep awake long enough to watch the news. I had no hope.

It was exciting to receive mail, and I had few visitors, being isolated and sick, I really wasn't up to it anyway. It was too far for my family to come for what would have been a very short visit.

Yes I did have a few sneaky visitors. The mother of the patient in the next room, who was having the same treatment for MS as I was, frequently popped in. She would like to see how I was getting on, and I communicated to her son through her. Our wall charts were compared, as well as our lives. One of the Doctors who was not directly involved in my case just sort of 'popped in' to see how I was. Another friend organized a visit from a Canberra based friend (who I had never met) to call in and see me. I can still see this poor woman trying to explain to the nurse that she needed to see me, although we had never met!

The second week of isolation wasn't much better. I watched the rain and wind outside but could not feel the breeze or smell the rain from inside. By day ten my blood count was on the move. My hemoglobin was 85, white cell count 0.6, platelets 7.0, neutrophils 0.56. I was on the mend. Diarrhea and nausea, as well as razor blade like indigestion plagued my day. Stool specimens and blood cultures were taken routinely, no cause found. I just had to ride it out. I still wonder at how I could be pouring out diarrhea at one end, and not being able to eat or hold anything down at the other? Mystery...

I was feeling crappy with nausea and diarrhea, but something else was happening. My MS hug, that first spasm of pain as you wake in the morning and start to stretch, was gone. The constant chronic pain in my hands had also disappeared. I was able for the first time in many years, lie in bed with my legs straight and not go into spasm with any small movement. The treatment had already begun to work. I was cautiously hopeful that I was on the road to recovery. Any small changes or improvements would be a bonus from here on in.

Well into week three, my blood count was rising towards normal. I could now shower and dress myself without having to stop and catch my breath. My room had become very small and I longed to be able to go outside and feel the breeze. All the isolation units have contained air-conditioning systems for reduced sources of infection, so the windows can't be opened. I would just have to wait. I was set to be discharged to my beloved high country the following week. Indigestion, nausea and diarrhea were still present, but manageable.

Late in week four, I set off with my surgical mask in place, to see the outside of the ward, and go to the hospital kiosk. I was desperate to get out of the unit and get a paper and some fresh juice. The nurses fitted me out in gown and mask and off I went. It's a fair hike to the kiosk, and I did have to stop and rest once on the way. I returned triumphant with sweets, juice and the paper. I was confident that I was improving in leaps and bounds, on track for discharge. It was only later that the nurses pointed out that I had walked all that way by myself, no walking stick! I had not even realized.

It wasn't all sunshine though. Over that weekend I developed a fever and begun having rigors. At this early stage, an infection is a real threat. Back to having daily blood cultures and specimen collections to track down any source of infection. I was seen by some infection specialists and commenced on the big gun antibiotics. No cause was found and the fever stopped after several days.

12.HOME

Finally ready for discharge! Five weeks later, I was ready to go home. Bed pressure on the acute unit was high, which is nothing new, so I was discharged to wait for Phill to pick me up to the Canberra Hospital residences overnight. The ward nurses came over to see that I was ok after I checked in. I was really touched to think they would do this for me. Remember we live 10hrs away, I had to wait for Phill to come to pick me up, then let him rest before we start back for home. I couldn't wait.

Phill hadn't seen me for over five weeks, so it was a bit of a shock when he arrived to pick me up. He wasn't sure that I was well enough for the long trip home. He kept saying 'You sure you're alright?'. I was twenty kilos lighter, very pale and weak, but all I wanted to do was get home. I hadn't been outside for a long time, so even though I was tired, I enjoyed the trip back. I wanted to hear Phill's voice and encouraged him to just talk, and fill in the gaps of what I had missed.

The seasons had already begun to change, and I felt that I had missed the summer. As we neared Guyra, I became quite emotional and began crying. I was so happy to be back. It was quite a special moment when we pulled up at home.

Not only was I emotionally overwhelmed, but physically as well. I had very little exercise tolerance and only made it from the front door to the back before being fatigued and having to stop and rest. I needed to realize my body needed time to repair and grow strong. I had to do things gradually, not an easy thing to do for me. In those first few weeks back I overdid things a fair bit, keen to see my friends and family and get my life back on track. At more than one time I was too breathless to speak, expecting my body to keep up with my plans for the day.

Physiotherapy and exercise, especially swimming, were a key to increasing strength. As I enjoy swimming, this wasn't really difficult. I could even get in and out of the pool now by myself. A really big step.

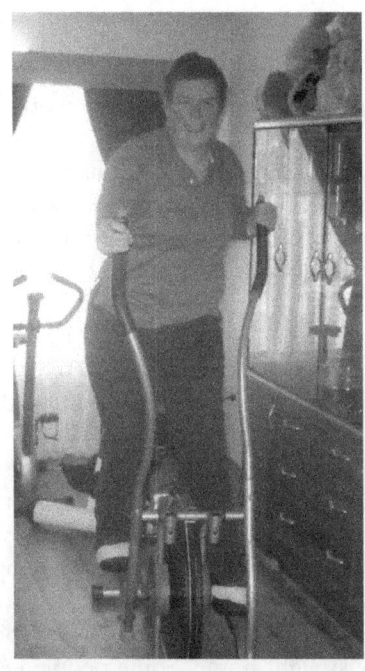

My hair began to regrow, and came back really soft and brown. I continued exercising and walking as far as I could each day to increase my muscle tone and strength. I was on no regular medications and my MS symptoms of muscular pain and spasms were much less.

Not one to rest on my laurels, I took my life back and started back volunteering at the Guyra St Vincent de Paul Centre, as well as The Hub, our local neighborhood center.

One year on, back to Canberra for my first yearly review. Good news, no new brain lesions and my disease was in remission. I was making steady progress with walking and distance, and chronic pain was a thing of the past. I will always have a residual limp in my left leg, but I am continually working on my gait to make walking more natural. Weakened muscles need a long time and hard work to regain function.

While in Canberra, I took the time to visit the apheresis unit to touch base and thank the staff who had helped me so much. It is good for the staff to see that their hard work does pay off. At that time there was a woman in the unit being harvested for stem cell transplant. I wished her luck in her journey. This particular patient would be the source of much controversy in the coming months. Her stem cells were harvested and frozen. Before they could be reinfused, the Canberra Ethics Committee had ceased the program. Imagine how devastated that poor person was to find out after all that build up and preparation that she was not going on for further treatment as planned. Subsequently, the transplant took place much later at a different facility, after much hard work and public outcry. See reference below for the story.

I was progressing along nicely, and had recommenced studying at TAFE, and even secured a part time job with accounts at the local neighborhood center. My mind fog and confusion gone, I was able to concentrate to study and work effectively. I was able to type two handed again (still can't spell).

Keeping in contact with Carmel Turner, I was always in awe of how Carmel got the message out there. Her web pages and comprehensive information and videos let people know that there was an effective treatment available.

For my part, to help get the message out, in late 2013 I agree to do an interview with Channel Seven's Today Tonight program. The reporter arranged for me to fly to Sydney for the interview. At that time we were caring for Phill's father, who has non-Hodgkin's lymphoma. Well family is a funny thing, one of Phill's sisters can't do enough to help us, but the other sister wouldn't care for her own father for the day. So I had to fly down, do the interview and fly straight home. Some people just can't be counted on. Anyway the interview went well and was widely shown.

https://www.youtube.com/watch?v=ozoKBN-6cNQ

The YouTube interview is titled: The Stem cell therapy delivering incredible results to MS sufferers.

I have also spoken at the local Rotary and Probus club, and I am very active in online forums and chats. A vast amount of information is out there online. I have also spoken and presented at the MS Support group that I first went to when I was diagnosed. It was in response to an inundation of comments in an online HSCT group that the seed for documenting my journey and writing this book was formed. There is so much need and so many people wanting this information.

As I have said before, the world doesn't stop turning when someone is having a crisis. While I was recovering, and building back my strength, my family suffered another crisis. My youngest son Robert was critically injured in a car accident. He was not expected to survive. His injuries were extensive, and it was a true test of all our strengths over that period when it was touch and go. Without the treatment that I had in Canberra, there would have been no way I would have been capable of being with my son, travelling to and forth to Newcastle, and staying by his side for weeks to see if he would recover. I just would not have been capable of doing it. Robert did survive, against all odds, and has made a miraculous recovery.

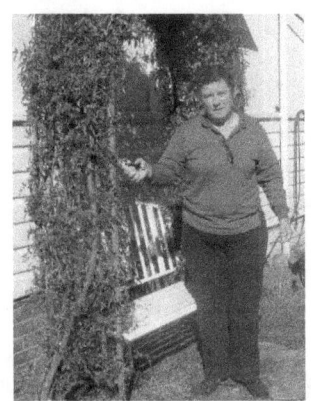

I attend a yearly review at Dr Colin J Andrews practice in Canberra, and am happy to report that I am better each year. I have no new brain lesions or symptoms. My medical records have been added to the national HSCT register that has been established. I no longer need my walking stick and can manage to walk independently anywhere I wish. I have no regular medications prescribed. I continue to work part time and study, as well as volunteer in my local community, and at the Guyra Community Garden, where I am a founding member. My family and friends are amazed at my recovery and I am still finding improvements in things that I can do, like typing a book..

I am in my third year of recovery post-transplant, and continue to see small improvements. Anyone considering 'rolling the dice' on this treatment needs to consider many factors. The main consideration for me was, did I want a life of chronic and debilitating pain, with the gradual loss of the use of my body, or would I strive to be well and regain my life if I could?

I have no regrets, as I sit here and type this diary of my journey. I don't reflect on where I would be now without the transplant, I look forward to a full and active happy life. I might go for a walk outside later….

Additional Information

This book was written from a patient perspective, it is a personal journey meant to be a guide only.

Please consult with experts in this specialty for medical advice

Not all types of MS can be successfully treated with this therapy.

Many online groups and forums have information and files on various overseas treatments available, currently over a dozen different countries offer this procedure. See Facebook and search for Hematopoietic Stem Cell Transplant to locate groups, or a simple google search.

For clinical trials in Australia related to HSCT, see *www.anzctr.org.au*